DATE DUE NOV 3 0 2005

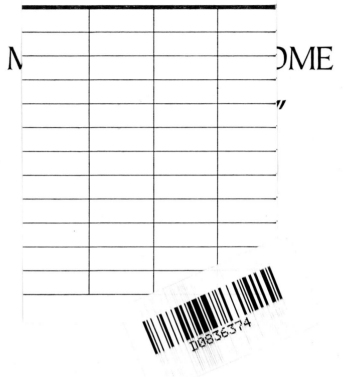

N   DME

"

MAKING YOUR HOME
"SENIOR-FRIENDLY"

A Guide for Friends and Family

by
Chuck Oakes

cp

AVENTINE PRESS

Published by Aventine Press
1023 4th Ave #204
San Diego CA, 92101
www.aventinepress.com

Library of Congress Cataloging-in-Publication Data
2004105707

ISBN: 1-59330-170-7

Table of Contents

Introduction
MAKING YOUR HOME *SENIOR-FRIENDLY*
A Guide for Family and Friends

The only constant in life is change! Life changes can be traumatic and difficult. Change of career, jobs, death of a loved one, serious medical problems and accidents can have serious consequences on one's plans for the future. As technology improves and lifespans increase due to improved health care and medical breakthroughs, we are faced with the reality that there is no escaping the fact that *"aging is what's happening!"*

As a baby-boomer with aging parents, who are still residing in the home we lovingly call *"The Oakes Homestead"*, I find myself doing what I can to make the autumn of their days as safe, secure and enjoyable as I can, for as long as I can. My brother and I were always encouraged to create, whether it is in the kitchen or in the family woodshop. Now that I *am 50-something*, I find myself enjoying the opportunity to collaborate with my parents as they face the challenges of aging. Yes, I do have my own life and career. Sometimes my work takes me away and someday I may have to relocate, but in the meantime I take advantage of the time available to be of assistance. Frankly, I enjoy the opportunity to create and develop new ideas and *"life enrichment techniques"* in making life safer and easier for my parents. This primer contains some ideas that I hope will prove inspirational and helpful to you and your family. It's all about quality of life.

In writing this information, I have emphasized **four key areas:**
 1. Safety
 2. Security
 3. Convenience
 4. Comfort

Although the focus and intent of this information was designed for aging parents, many of the concepts and suggestions could be applied to loved ones of any age with limited abilities.

Certain assumptions have been made in the development of this material. If your loved one has medical, physical or mental "challenges", the modifications and home-delivered-services are therefore customized to suit the particular deficiency or challenge. The suggestions contained herein should make life easier for everyone.... of all ages!

The intent of this primer is to inspire and enlighten readers with the understanding that support of your aging parents includes consultations with experts in financial, insurance and medical matters.

Assuming that your parents are well enough to communicate normally, it is best to begin to explore the topic of *their future* in a comfortable setting and time. Have an open mind as you introduce the idea of their future needs and desires. Try to ascertain *the perceptions* of your parents. Realize that they may not be receptive to your input and assistance at first. Be patient. They may also be reluctant to accept your ideas of forming a committee-type process in managing their welfare when for many years, there was no need for such intervention. You will notice their reluctance to change. That's OK. Don't be surprised if they prefer to stay with an *incompetent* landscaper, financial planner or housekeeper to avoid something new and unfamiliar. Watch for *signs of stress* and a sense of being *overwhelmed* such as tears and obvious distress. **Learn to back off and to be sensitive to their needs and level of comfort.**

"Reality Check"

Give your parents the *space and dignity* to be themselves! They are valued; they have ideas, perceptions and preferences, even if their capabilities and faculties are somewhat diminished. Be patient with them. I have found that I sometimes respond and react to them *as if* they were much younger, they are not. While this may seem rather insensitive, you have to be mindful of the reality of the moment. Let's not confuse mental with physical impairments. Chances are that they are *more* frustrated than you are with their disabilities and aging bodies. Give them time, patience, respect and the courtesy they deserve. With the space and respect they deserve, allow them "veto power" over the new ideas and recommendations you may offer.

A word of caution:
"The Dragon Slayer Syndrome"

As I assist my parents in their home, I notice that I occasionally act as a *slayer of dragons*. My role as a caregiver and son can evolve into an obsessive problem solver...a *dragon slayer* of sorts...if I am not careful. It is all about *choice*...and not simply problem solving! Sometimes the mission is not so much to "fix" but rather to "feel". That is, to express concern and love for your parents by *really listening* might be just what is needed and appreciated....rather than always striving to *repair, fix or handle*. If your parents possess the abilities to make decisions and use sound judgement ...great, give them the space and opportunity to do so. In a caregiver mode, you must maintain the ability to assess their abilities while providing what is needed. As you will find out, if you haven't already, maintaining the "status quo" is convenient and comfortable for many seniors.

The other day, my parents and I were discussing the never-ending struggle of both the birds and squirrels in their search for food during the winter. We are committed to assisting both birds and squirrels by supplying corn and feed. As you might have experienced, the struggle becomes a real challenge as to who gets the most food. Word spreads throughout the neighborhood and suddenly the entire squirrel population finds your feeders. This escalation of a helpful deed turns into a stressful and potentially dangerous situation in that the feeders are situated above snow and ice, making it impossible for my parents to *safely* maintain. You get the picture. We spend a great deal of time on how we can satisfy both squirrels and birds while keeping safe from falling on the ice and snow. Yes, we utilize squirrel proof feeders. After several minutes of focussing on the danger of my Dad or Mom attempting to fill the feeders, or chase the critters, I lost my sensitivity and told them that our apparent obsession with feeding the animals was, in the grand scheme of things, inconsequential and rather insignificant! I later realized my tactless outburst and explained to them that in the choice between safety and feeding the critters....the obvious choice is always safety! However, I realized that in my outburst, I was telling them that what was entertaining and fun for them was insignificant. What right does anyone have to tell *you* that what you value is insignificant? We strive to satisfy all the outside creatures while attending to the safety and interests of our parents.

The rising cost of caregiving in the workplace:

As a member of the "sandwich generation" (individuals who take care of their own children while supporting and assisting aging parents), Baby Boomers are under pressure to perform at work while doing all the supportive tasks needed by both generations. The *annual cost* to employers of workers taking care of *parents* is increasing[1]—

- Absenteeism: $397 million
- Partial absenteeism: $488 million
- Workday interruptions: $3.7 billion
- Eldercare crises: $1 billion
- Costs associated with supervising caregivers: $805 million
- Annual replacement costs for employees who quit: $4.9 billion
- Lost productivity: $11.4 to $29 billion

As family caregivers, what are we supposed to do? What can we do?

The challenge of supporting aging parents can be difficult and daunting. This primer offers suggestions and helpful hints on perspectives, resources and devices that can enable you to maintain your own life and career while supporting your parents in their own home. Utilizing some of the ideas contained herein can help minimize the adverse impact of caregiving.

What can employers do?

Commit to a corporate support strategy that provides the information and opportunity for employees to help their aging loved ones.

Disclaimer

The reader agrees to indemnify, defend, and hold harmless Chuck Oakes (the Author) from any and all liability, penalties, losses, damages, costs, expenses, attorneys' fees, causes of action or claims caused by or resulting indirectly from your application or use of the suggestions provided in this text which damages either you, or any other party or parties without limitation or exception. This indemnification and hold harmless agreement extends to all issues associated with your purchase of this text and any and all materials associated with it.

Chapter One
Take Care of Yourself

As your family's caregiver, the first thing to re-member is that changes aren't always convenient, easy and comfortable. Patience and realistic expectations are needed. So, take a deep breath and remind yourself that you're doing the right thing and you can make a difference!

Do what we can, with what we've got....while we've got it! It is essential to remember that your effectiveness, success and endurance through this process of supporting your parents rely heavily on your own maintenance, health and energy. If you don't take care of yourself.... you cannot expect to take care of others! Manage and maintain a high level of enthusiasm and energy.

Realize your limitations & resources

Time, money, energy, abilities, etc. are sometimes in limited supply. Take stock of your available resources before plunging ahead!

Some suggestions for caregivers:

- Eat and sleep enough
- Set realistic personal goals
- Take up a hobby or enjoy a sport
- Love and laugh more often
- Stay connected to others
- Join a support group or association (see chapter on Resources)
- Be kind to yourself- do something *for you!*
- The use of lists and reminder boards are invaluable for everyone to maintain control of their hectic lives and busy schedules. The day I won my Palm Pilot was a day I will never forget! From that time forward, I am actually keeping on top of things and remembering a lot more than I did without it. However, if you use such a personal management device, you must backup to your home PC regularly.

Give your parents the space and dignity to be themselves. They still have valuable ideas, perceptions and preferences...although their physical and mental abilities may be somewhat diminished. Be patient with yourself and with them. I have found that it is automatic to respond and to react to them as if they were much younger, when they are not. While we all age at different speeds and degrees, we should remind ourselves that life and capabilities change as we age.

Chapter Two

Expectations, Assessments and Perceptions

You may be *ready* to support your loved ones, but are you *prepared*?

Accept and affirm

We all need acceptance and affirmation that we are worth something to someone. Especially with seniors, it is important to recognize their present as well as their past value. Seniors represent a family heritage, value system and memories. Many cultures throughout the world embrace and celebrate their aging relatives and ancestors...however, all too often, we tend to forget and discard people who are not in the mainstream of American society. (Seniors and citizens with disabilities are two groups who fall into this category all too often.) Take time to reaffirm their worth to you and your family.

Needs Assessment- Perception or Reality?

- What are the perceived vs. actual needs of your parents?
- For instance, does Mom actually have a hearing problem, or is it a case of selective hearing?
- Focus on "abilities", not "disabilities"! Strive to satisfy or enhance the interests of your loved ones consistent with their abilities.
- Evaluate the condition of the home. Is it in need of repairs, if so, how extensive?
- What steps have been (or should be) developed to address these repairs?

Establish a list of priorities that concentrate on security, safety, convenience and comfort.

- Who does the cleaning and how often?
- Who and how are these chores to be completed?
- What chores or duties are being avoided or neglected?
- How well do your parents care for themselves in terms of their hygiene, appearance, fitness and health?

Objects of Obligation

In our dedication, support and love, we tend to focus on the duties, chores and responsibilities associated with providing service to our senior loved ones. The problem often develops that this hard work can come across as *obligation and not desire.* Remind them and yourself that there are other (perhaps more important) aspects of support they need...your time, love and caring...rather than doing, building or other active participation. *Being with* or *"doing for"* someone is the question.

Taking Stock of the Capabilities of Your Parents

Physical Challenges
Communication Challenges/ Hearing Loss

It is interesting and coincidental that when my Dad had his hearing checked, it was found that the lost frequencies were identical to those of my Mom's voice! What a coincidence! The higher end of the sound spectrum is usually that used by women. Of course, my Dad says he has mastered the *art and science* of selective hearing (!) When he selects to use his hearing aid (high frequency loss has been confirmed), he now speaks so softly that my Mother cannot hear him. Yet, another challenge. I initiated discussion of the value and benefit of "staying in touch" with one another, as if I had to remind them after 61 years of wedded bliss! It is a blessing that they have one another. However, when communication breaks down....the connection between them can suffer. I tactfully remind my Dad occasionally that when he does NOT utilize his hearing aids, distance is formed between Mom and him. **When you are "not connected" you become "disconnected"!** I have also noticed how the family members sometimes exclude our Dad from conversations when he fails to use his hearing device and misinterprets conversation. In this way, it is easy to understand how people can misinterpret a hearing impaired individual as one of limited mental ability, rather than simply with a hearing impairment.

It is important to realize that everyone is unique and may experience hearing loss differently. Therefore, have your parents' hearing checked to find out definitely what they are experiencing. My Dad has lost his higher frequencies, others I have spoken with have lost their low-end sounds.   With the advancement of digital hearing devices, there are many places that offer free hearing tests.   That is where I went to get my hearing checked…with my Dad as a "witness".

Some tips:
* Reinforce the concept that every family member plays a role in the support of your parents.   That is, Dad and Mom should not have unrealistic expectations when talking with one another.   Regardless of the use of a hearing enhancement device or not, you should try to speak to your parent in the same room and preferably, in front of them.
* Also, try to speak more distinctly and slowly…not necessarily loudly but perhaps in a slightly lower register, depending upon the frequency loss.

Flavorless Foods and Aromas

My parents and I have noticed that foods and aromas don't seem as strong as they used to be.   When you think of it, isn't it reasonable to expect sensory cells to age along with the rest of us?   Consequently, don't always blame the grocer or butcher for *less-than-flavorful* food. Therefore, you might consider choosing stronger candles or using more vibrant spices to enhance your meals. (more later on this topic) Certain mild foods might require some enhancing and embellishment with herbs and sauces.

Suggestion: Try using a crock-pot, or other slow cooker to enhance flavor and tenderness of food. These cookers can make food preparation easier.

Potential danger—
With our abilities to smell diminish, so are abilities to *detect* spoiled foods. Keep this in mind when you visit your parents. Check out the refrigerator for outdated milk, moldy cheese, etc.

Multiple *"Challenges"*

My parents are well suited for each other, thank goodness. My Dad is a retired mechanical engineer and my Mom is a retired Hooker...*of rugs*! They compliment each other nicely. One is creative and aesthetic while the other is practical and structural.

Extremely proficient in her craft, Mom was one of the founders of the **Association of Traditional Hooking**

Artists, A.T.H.A. She is extremely creative and, of course, visual. However, she is now experiencing difficulty in walking and has accepted the benefits of using a cane or walker for support. She is also suffering with a vision condition known as *macular degeneration*. As you can imagine, it is extremely tiring for her to cope with both mobility and visual problems, especially when so much of her life has revolved around the ability to get around and to see. It can be daunting and challenging, to say the least! Fortunately, she will not be blind, according to the specialists, although we always hope for improvement. For many seniors, multiple disabilities present constant frustration and sometimes depression. My "dragon-slayer" tendency is to reinforce the abilities she still possesses, when in reality, she may tire of my "constant positive attitude" in my attempts to rectify or correct her problems. I have since learned to step back and reflect before responding rather than immediately reacting to the particular challenge of the moment.

"Step back and reflect before responding"

Team Work is Essential

As a team, the family must work together in supporting the aging family members. Sharing the chores and responsibilities is very important although not always practical when distances are involved. When living with a person with disabilities, it is critical to be sensitive to both disabilities and abilities. Caregivers and companions need to be careful not to make assumptions and to be realistic in their expectations. For instance, you can't expect a hearing impaired individual to clearly hear and understand conversation *outside* of the room. This is unrealistic, even with the use of hearing aids or devices.

Quality of Life Means Having Some *Fun*

Aging gracefully can have its benefits. More time and fewer responsibilities leave time for family, friends and hobbies. As a nation, we are living longer and spending more time away from our employment than ever before. Now the challenge is "time management", i.e. what to do with all the free time. As a caregiver of aging parents, you should realize the importance of social affiliations, hobbies and crafts. They all have their benefits to the individual and family. They contribute to stress management and overall quality of life. We are living longer now, let's build in some fun and adventure as we age!

Some suggestions: (Depending upon the abilities and interests of your parents.)

1. Day trips (other than to the doctor or grocery store).
2. Activities at the local Senior Center.
3. Special meals outside of the home.
4. Courses of special interest at the local community college or Senior Center.
5. Encourage outside interests, hobbies and crafts.

Pets and Plants (We all need to be needed)

Taking care of "living" things can be highly pleasurable and can offer some nice benefits. There is a technique known as "pet therapy" which has evolved due to the intrinsic and therapeutic benefits of taking care of something living that responds to your care and attention. Plants and especially pets offer unconditional love and acceptance, something we all can use! For many years, my family enjoyed various kinds of pets, including chickens, parakeets, dogs and fish. However, as times change, so does the feasibility of taking care of pets and plants. My Mom and Dad now take care of many plants but I must admit that the *silk ones* are the most "user-friendly"!

Word of caution: choose the plant or pet wisely, according to the level of care and maintenance required. You wouldn't want to add burden or undue responsibility to someone with limited capability. Match the level of care required to the abilities of the owner.

Social Affiliations
If you don't participate...you stagnate!

Social affiliations are important, including church activities, sports, crafts, etc. Volunteer opportunities are great to build self-worth and reduce stress. (If you want to feel better about yourself.... do something for someone else, especially when they least expect it!) Participation on committees can help as long as the responsibilities don't become stressful or too taxing. However, when mobility becomes a problem and your parents are no longer driving themselves, it's time to identify local resources. Taxis and town shuttles are two obvious sources. Also, there are neighbors and friends who might really enjoy providing occasional assistance. Churches and their affiliates can also be a source of volunteers and assistance. When boredom sets in, it's time to be creative. Depending upon financial resources, inviting friends and family members for an afternoon tea might be an appropriate and not-too-taxing or stressful event. It need not be fancy or elaborate. Many retirement communities provide shuttle service for their residents, as do many towns. Friends of your parents could be driven to the party. The event could be at a local restaurant or in your home. Like people of all ages, many seniors hesitate to reach out to neighbors, either for help or to express concern. Somehow, there is always an excuse or explanation why the outreach is inconvenient or uncomfortable. In actuality, the *mere act* of calling a neighbor to find out how they are doing is beneficial and can relieve stress. Take the initiative to make a difference in someone else's life!

Don't Impose *YOUR* life onto Theirs!

You might feel that your parent's lifestyle is boring and incomplete. Don't be too quick to judge and react. Their lifestyle and activity level may be perfectly suited for *their interests and capabilities.* Their weekly activities are theirs, not yours. Activities may revolve around doctor visits and shopping, but hopefully include a variety of other experiences. I've learned with my parents that grocery shopping can be a viable *social activity* where they meet neighbors and friends. Their shopping excursions are not only needed for groceries, but also provide exercise. Ideally, they will engage in some social connections and affiliations, but these affiliations and activities should be enjoyable and rewarding. Otherwise, encourage them to evaluate their participation.

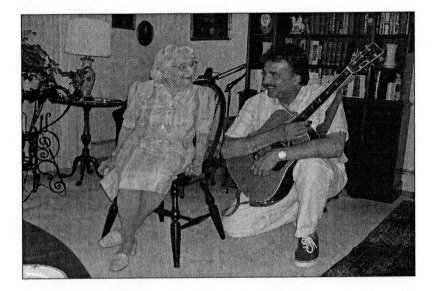

Phone calls, visits and the importance of reliability

Nothing is more aggravating to seniors than last minute change of plans. Realizing that everyone reacts differently to the same situations, visits and trips are something to anticipate and to plan for. Hence, when these plans are changed, it can be very disappointing. Visits and phone calls can be very special moments; therefore we should make every effort to understand their value to our loved ones. When you say you will visit on a particular day and time, be there! Honor your commitment. As with others of any age, don't over-promise and under-deliver! When siblings are available, share the load....share the responsibility of supporting the parents.

Phone calls can be really important, especially as sociability decreases with those outside the home. Consider calling your parents on a regular, routine schedule if possible. This keeps everyone connected and current. Some church and community groups have a support *hotline* arrangement whereby someone calls at the same scheduled time daily. If there is no answer, emergency services are contacted to investigate.

Depression and Related Challenges

During the journey with your loved ones, it is essential that you develop and practice effective communication skills, especially when there are hearing problems or speech deficiency involved. As you communicate with your parents, remind yourself of the specific challenges and conditions with which they cope. Be patient, deliberate and communicate at a pace *they can understand* and keep up with. Be patient and kind in repeating messages to them. (I have found myself raising my voice when they don't understand something.... sometimes, it is volume, other times, it is simply the rapid delivery! Instead of fast-food....it's *fast-speak*!) As you assist them and help them maintaining their home, (to whatever extent you can), remember to visit occasionally with NO CHORES to perform. They don't want to become obligations or chores to their family members. Whenever possible, try to include them in whatever you're doing, as appropriate. For example, I customized a teacart (more on this later) recently in the family workshop and invited my Dad to participate to whatever extent HE chose. We found that the experience working together was therapeutic for both of us and brought back fond memories of our past.

Signs of depression include irritability, excess drinking or eating, sleeping disorders, emotional roller coaster, drastic weight gain or loss. Of course, many symptoms are difficult to diagnose at this stage of life, hence, bring in the specialists if you are concerned. **Stay in tune and in touch** with your parents. Support, love and assist…but respect their relative competencies and existing faculties. Allow them to participate in life in the manner in which they are still able to do so. I have learned that **CHANGE is a real problem** and it manifests itself in various ways. For instance, making a date for a future visit is important for most seniors; it gives them something to anticipate and look forward to. For some, however, it causes stress and anxiety…. when this happens, advance notice may not be the best practice.

Outside Assistance and Resources

Our country's health industry is undergoing continued revision and revamping. For the sake of your sanity and your parents' wellness and health support, locate your local Department of Geriatrics or Department of Aging. These organizations can be excellent resources for information and services in your town. Towns often have Geriatric Social Workers available for residents. Be advised that these specialists may be affiliated with a university hospital. The university affiliation sometimes takes some getting used to. For instance, you may rarely see your designated physician, but rather an intern ...and that may vary each visit.

Ultimately, if your parents continue to reside at home, they will need some assistance, whether medical and health related or some other support. Outside assistance can present security issues for your family. One of the benefits of working through agencies for help is that the people coming onto your property will be bonded and you will have some course of action against the agency should something be broken or damaged. If you don't use an agency, you are on your own and should do the reference checking yourself.

Anticipate resistance from your loved ones if you have to make personnel changes in household helpers. Remember that CHANGE causes discomfort and distress. For someone with limited visibility, the scratches on their beautiful cherry furniture or the broken outside patio table leg may be overlooked. Be tactful, sensitive and patient.

Medication, Doctors and Healthcare Monitoring

The healthcare, insurance and medical industries are changing daily. For seniors, taking care of their wellness, health and medications can be a daunting task. Consequently, it is beneficial for the families of seniors to take an active role in the management of care for their parents. If possible, accompany them on visits to their doctors. Going with them will bolster their confidence and show them you care. Also, it shows the doctors that you are there and taking an active caregiver's role. As a caregiver, keep records of doctors' names and contact information for your files. I keep records of current medications for both parents and ask them to update them periodically. I also provide daily medication worksheets and a folder for my parents to maintain a record for taking drugs. Pharmacies usually carry pill dispensers in weekly and monthly arrangements. These can be very handy.

Chapter Three

Room by Room

The Home Itself -The *Basic Checklist*[2]
As we explore sections of the home, we remind ourselves of our mission and specific criteria:
1. Safety
2. Security
3. Comfort
4. Convenience

Specific devices and gadgets are described in Chapter Five.

*   *   *   *

You may be thinking of **adding onto your home with an apartment** for Mom or Dad. If you are, you're not alone. Many families consider this option to support their aging parents. There are many considerations when families think about having loved ones join them in their homes, especially when they have limited abilities. You should plan for their future needs as well as those they have today.

Some of the concerns and considerations include:

- Financial
- Abilities/disabilities of the new resident-present and anticipated
- Town zoning regulations and appropriate codes
- Tax deductions
- Qualified contractors

Your lifestyle and that of your parent(s) should be taken into account as you move together. Some of the suggestions here are structural and should be discussed with the contractor, builder or architect prior to construction. Other items and devices can be installed after construction to an existing or new home. Some of the ***structural items*** include:

- Thresholds no more than ½" high
- Doorways no less than 36" wide[3]
- Intercom and stereo sound system throughout the house

Kitchen

- Under-the-counter lighting
- Consider having the height of the cabinets 15" rather than the standard 18-24"; making it easier to reach items

Other Ideas
- Automated emergency lighting
- Optional house generator in event of power outage
- Locks and doors
- Door levers rather than door knobs
- Grab rails and grab bars in the bathroom, stairways and entryways

The Layout of the Residence (apartment, house or condo)

It is important to have a layout that is senior-friendly and safe. The suggestions in the following chapters will assist you in exploring ways to improve the safety and comfort of various rooms.

Suggestions:
- Ground floor living area
- Bathroom proximity to the bedroom

Although my parents have not had to experience *major* renovations, we have implemented many of the following items listed below.

Entrance area
Motion Detectors to Activate Lighting
(see Chapter Five)

My family has several outside motion detectors that activate lighting units. Two detectors light the front entryway and two light the rear entry to the "Oakes Homestead". They are fabulous for safety and convenience. The porch unit utilizes the external sensor unit with the screw-in bulb connector that goes right into the bulb area of the lighting fixture. It works great. A surveillance camera system is worth considering for special needs or circumstances.

Consider the following as you walk around:
- Condition of sidewalk and entryway.
- Peephole in doorway.
- Is a ramp needed?
- Would grabrails or hand holds help?
- Are the door locks easy to operate and lock?
- Are handles or levers used?
- Is it easy and convenient to get the mail?
- Doorbells/chimes loud enough to be heard throughout the residence. They can be wireless with multiple chime units.

Walkways and Paths

Of course, an entry ramp is essential for those requiring a wheelchair. Maintain a smooth and level approach to your entryway. Flagstone and other stones can change after a winter freeze; hence, be sure to maintain them to ensure safe entry. Think about replacing them with level Walkways made from poured cement or molded stones from concrete. Railings and handholds are valuable also. (See Chapter Five)

Living Room

- Chairs and sofas....are they easy to get in and out of?
  Chairs can provide support throughout the home. However, in the case of visual impairment, they can be tripping hazards. Be sensitive as to the placement of furniture.
- Are carpets secured and flat? Do they need to be retacked?
- Is the lighting sufficient for the purpose needed? (Indirect, subtle, bright for craft work and reading, etc.)
- Candles and lanterns away from flammable objects.
- Have the sofa and chairs been thoroughly cleaned

and/or vacuumed? (To reduce dirt, dander, dust, mites and related allergens.)

Kitchen

- Adequate lights for activated stove and oven. (Can these lights be readily seen to prevent leaving them ON?)
- Under-the-counter lighting is especially helpful for the visually impaired in order to avoid accidents.
- Hazardous material safely stored.
- Are appliance cords out of the way?
- Are the appliances easy to read and use?
- "Lazy-Susans" in corner cabinets can help access goods. Cupboards should be easy to reach and store items.
- Rounded knobs on cabinets rather than those that can catch clothing.
- Door latches that work and close securely.
- Allow for a sitting area to rest in the kitchen, perhaps allowing for a chair to go under the counter somewhere and the countertop at a comfortable height.
- Step stool that has handholds.
- Extension "grab arm" to reach high things on shelves.
- Shelves that come out to you rather than having to reach into them.

Bathroom

The majority of injuries are from trips and falls; many in the bathroom.

There are numerous enhancements for people with limited mobility. Here are some ideas to consider:

- Grabrails and handholds inside the tub area and elsewhere in the room, as needed.
- Heat lamp in ceiling with fan.
- Avoid throw rugs, but if used, make certain they are secured with non-skid backing.
- Emergency communication device (if there is one resident, a phone is a good idea or other emergency device for contacting police or ambulance. If there are other residents, a simple handbell will alert others within the home).
- Would an elevated, high-rise toilet seat help?
- Shower or bath? What improvements might be needed?
- Seat in tub, either permanent or temporary.
- Shower wand (makes directing the water much easier and will enable the individual to sit while showering).
- Are medications easy to find and use? (Discard outdated medications.)

- Non-skid mats or strips inside the tub.
- Guardrails inside the tub/shower (secured to the studs if possible).
- Suitable lighting (in some applications, a wall-mounted motion detector to activate light can help).

Note: If a motion detector is used in the bathroom in the *wrong location*, it will shut itself off if it does not detect your presence while you are still "*busy*".

- Automating a light outside the bathroom entry is very handy for middle-of-the-night bathroom "*visits*". It can also serve as a security alert.
- Specialized lift equipment is available for those needing assistance in accessing the tub and shower area.

Bedroom
- Lights that are easy to activate at night with controls located at the bedside.
- Device to notify family/emergency services in event of a fall.
- Automated lighting inside closets.
- Smoke and carbon monoxide detectors.
- Is the phone readily available? (Cell phone, cordless or regular.)

- Is there emergency lighting installed or available? (In event of power failure.)
- Flashlights with batteries.
- Is the bed in good shape?

  The height of the bed should be appropriate for the resident. There are mattresses and box springs to suit every ability. For instance, a lower bed will better enable a senior to get into and out of bed but this also depends upon the height of the individual. A bed that is too close to the floor is difficult to get up from. A tall person would feel more comfortable with a higher bed than a shorter person would.
- Night lights. (Either the ones that come on at night and off in the morning, or those that are activated by motion.)

Whole Home Considerations

Telephones

- How many phones in use?
- Is there at least *one permanent* phone available? (Cordless phones may not work in power outages.)
- Is there a message machine/service in use? Is it easy to use?

- Would special phones be helpful for the hearing impaired? (For example, phones with blinking light, amplifiers or speakerphones.)
- Phones with pictures can help dial numbers quickly and easily.

Fireplaces and Woodstoves

My family really loves fireplaces and woodstoves. There are many considerations for the enjoyment of fireplaces and woodstoves. As we have emphasized, always remember the capabilities of the residents. The options include:

- Propane fireplaces (some with remote controls)
- Manufactured fireplace logs (These are made from wood ingredients and many are advertised to burn cleaner than real wood)
- Wood pellets (for woodstoves)

In front of our fireplace, we have a glass door and screen for protection against flying sparks. The glass door reduces heat loss up the chimney. Because we enjoy the ambiance of wood burning, due diligence is appropriate to prevent accidents. Here are some reminders:

- Chimney repair and maintenance

When was the most recent time it was inspected and cleaned? A professional should check the chimney once a year.

- The process of starting the fire. Can your parents do this safely? If not, consider a propane wireless controlled unit that can start and stop the fire with the push of a button!
- Fire extinguishers can save lives...keep them handy!
- Handheld fire-starters fueled by lighter fluid can often be safer to use than matches. Again, evaluate the abilities and comfort of your parents.

Water heater temperature should be below 120 degrees F to prevent scalding.

Extension cords Are there too many? Are the wires, cords and plugs in good condition?

If space heaters are used, are they properly located to prevent being knocked over?

In Event of Emergency (more in Chapter Four)

Emergencies can occur anywhere in the home. Therefore, the use of detection and communication devices should be used throughout.

- Handheld communication device to call police or other emergency services in event of fall or injury.
- Smoke, fire and chemical/radon/carbon monoxide detectors (some automatically contact police when activated).

Medical information should be summarized and accessible to emergency personnel in event of an emergency. Each town has its own preference on where to store such information. Some towns ask that a medical summary be placed inside the refrigerator in a container, while other towns ask that the information be attached outside the refrigerator in a folder. Some towns recommend an outside light or insignia to better enable emergency personnel to find your home.

Inside Air Quality

Maintaining healthy air quality in any home can be challenging but essential for a safe and friendly home.

Air Purification

Several options for air purification:
- **Ozone producing units** for treating the air in a room or entire house. When used properly, ozone can be

used effectively to purify and cleanse pools and the air in a home or work environment without the use of chemicals. The units I have used can be adjusted to produce the right amount of cleansing ozone.

- **Ionic purification units** to treat and cleanse the air in a room. They frequently utilize a filter (see below) to capture dirty air. Carbon filters are also frequently included with these units to enhance air cleansing.

- **HEPA (High Efficiency Particulate Air) filtration units** are frequently included with Ionic purifiers because they are superb at capturing particles in the air. These filters must be replaced and can be expensive.

- **Electronically charged metal plates** attract pollutants within a house and can be easily washed off without expensive filters to replace. The units can be rather expensive but do NOT require a filter, hence, some cost savings in terms of routine maintenance.

In Chapter Seven we discuss the benefits of plants in the home as natural air purifiers.

Vacuum cleaners

The purchase of an effective vacuum cleaner can improve the quality of the home air. Before replacing my own vacuum cleaner, I did some research into the latest and most effective vacuum cleaners. I used *Consumer Reports* as my reference. One of the criteria, that was important for my family and me was HEPA filtration. The HEPA filtration system is used in air purifiers and vacuum cleaners. In vacuums, the filters reduce the dust and dirt from being blown around the room as you vacuum. Make sure to replace the vacuum bags and check the filters in your vacuum cleaner regularly.

Filters to Check and Replace Regularly

When considering the air quality of a home, there are factors to evaluate, including the ease and cost of replacement filters. It's best to review the *Consumer Reports* or other resources for the latest evaluation. It is easy to forget, but the maintenance of home filters can make a huge difference in the quality and health of living at home. I remind myself to check all the filters in my parents home regularly, some more frequently than others, "To help me remember to change filters, etc., I rely on my Palm Pilot…a great help." These filters include:

- Furnace filters
- Water filters in the kitchen but also whole-house filters, if used.

- Humidifiers
- Air purifiers
- Vacuum filters and replacement of bags

In hot air heating systems, it is essential to have the vents and ductwork of the house *cleaned and disinfected* every couple of years.

Don't Forget to Check Batteries!

When I am checking and replacing the filters in the home, I check and replace batteries while I'm at it. Consider checking the following:

- Television and VCR remote control units
- Wireless doorbells (both doorbell button and the chime units)
- Wireless temperature and humidity gauges
- Garage door openers
- All fire, smoke and carbon monoxide alarm units
- Flashlights and emergency lighting

Air Humidity Levels

A healthy range of humidity in a home is between 35-50%. Homes that are below or above this healthy humidity range become more vulnerable to the flu virus. In the bedroom, I use a small humidifier and air purifier connected to timers for automatic activation before bedtime. I feel that cleaning the air prior to sleeping can improve the quality of sleep. While this doesn't guarantee a sound sleep, I think it helps. Don't forget to purchase a couple of gauges to monitor the humidity levels in the home.

When it comes to humidifiers, be careful that some whole-house units have a water reservoir in which a belt or wheel soaks up the water that eventually gets dispersed throughout the home. Reservoirs in either these whole-house units or in individual room humidifiers can breed bacteria. Therefore, if your humidifiers use reservoirs to hold the water, clean them with white vinegar regularly. Additives are available to add to the water that reduces the bacteria. However, these additives are not a substitute for regular cleaning. The manufacturer also will recommend a cleaner that is suited for your unit. The Oakes Homestead has three individual units plus a whole-house humidifier to maintain 40% humidity. I was unable to achieve and maintain a healthy humidity level with the whole-house unit alone.

Chapter Four

Emergency and Security Matters

Without becoming paranoid, there are some simple precautions and steps you can take to make your home more secure and safe from intruders. Most criminals know about home security systems and most do not want a "Gunfight at OK Corral" in your living room. While it is helpful to make the home look lived-in and occupied, criminals realize that people use timers and security systems. Today, you want to project the image that you CARE about your home and maintain a secure property. This attention includes security systems (whether simple or complex) and devices to make the home look cared-for and protected. For instance, too many people leave their homes unattended and vacant-looking. Due to frequent false alarms, some police departments and communities have mixed feelings about automated home security systems.

Here are some **common-sense tips** to consider:

Timers (See also Chapter Five)

It's best to purchase timers that vary the on and off times automatically. This variance enhances the "lived-in" appearance of your home. Place these timers out of sight, perhaps an upstairs bedroom so that no one can peer into the window to verify someone is actually home...or not.

- For lights
- For televisions and radios (to give the impression that someone is in the home)
- Automatic lighting (automatic on and off as the sun rises and sets)
- Plant a flower...Reduce Crime! (see Chapter Seven)

  As the President of our condo association, I often met with the local Police Services Department for updates on crime prevention and community auditing. I invited the Police Services Representative to audit our community for security and safety. At one of our meetings, we discussed how communities that look well maintained give the impression that they are also safe and secure. The Police mentioned how gardens and flowers enhance the beauty and security of a community.

- Avoid leaving newspapers or mail outside the home.
- Some communities encourage the establishment of Block Watch associations to improve and maintain security in a neighborhood.
- Have an empty dog dish outside.
- Using "beware of dog" signs can help.
- Tell a neighbor if you leave for any amount of time. Have neighbors tell you and/or your parents if they leave for extended periods of time.
- Give a neighbor a key to the home in the event emergency entry is needed by Police or Fire Departments.
- Motion detector lights are handy for you and for security.
- Security system *signs* alone can be a deterrent.
- Motion detector alarms/bells announce the arrival of someone approaching your home.

Emergency Kits for the Home[4]

With today's global uncertainty and insecurity, every home should be prepared for emergency. The following items should be included:

- First-Aid kit

- Food enough for 3-5 days (canned meats, fruits and vegetables)
- Water (one gallon per day per person; stored in plastic containers or bottled water)
- Soap
- Toilet paper
- Signal flares
- Shut-off wrench for house gas and water
- Plastic garbage bags
- Bleach
- Liquid detergent
- Fire extinguisher
- Paper and pencil
- Money/cash
- Batteries
- Flashlights
- Battery operated radio
- Candles (Depending upon the abilities of your parents, kerosene/oil lanterns and candles can be dangerous. Because they both require fire, they are not my choice for safe lighting in emergencies.)
- Battery-operated lanterns (some are rechargeable)

In Event of An Emergency, Do You Know Who to Call?

- Share emergency contacts information with family members
- Consider videotaping your parents or loved ones describing the location of important documents and other essential information. While you've got the camcorder available, I suggest recording the entire home for insurance purposes. In event of theft or fire, insurance companies will welcome a recording verifying home contents.
- Make a summary of key contacts for future reference and update it as needed. Such information should include:
- Attorney
- Accountant
- Phones numbers of close friends and family members
- Bank accounts
- Safe deposit boxes
- Insurance company and agent
- Location of important documents (in and outside your home)

Compiling a *Friends & Family* Roster

Speaking of making lists and gathering information, here's a story—

As you may recall, my Mom has Macular Degeneration that compromises her vision. So this holiday season, I customized a holiday greeting card for my parents to send out. I included a recent photo of them and on half of the cards, I included a note from my parents to the recipient. The initial process was tedious but well worth it. The customized approach with picture made it really special for people out of town. The large font made it easy to read.

Another added bonus of a master listing of family and friends is that it can help you to contact important people in event of a death or other major family change.

Life Alert (1-800-336-4415) Monitoring and Communication Devices and Systems

Perhaps you are aware of the buttons and bracelets that can be worn and activated easily in event of an emergency. The buttons and bracelets are connected to a master box in your home that can connect via a phone line to a central communication control center. I have just been updated that these systems can include a special emergency cell phone and the master monitoring box can actually enable emergency personnel to listen in on suspicious visitors at your home. Also, caregivers can monitor the home from a distance through an access code via the phone. The master monitoring box can also monitor movement. For instance, if your Mom is living alone and you reside 1,000 miles distant and you travel frequently, the box will actually monitor the *movement* within the house and if there is none in a specified period of time, it activates emergency communication! In my opinion, this is a welcome advance in emergency assistance and response.

Chapter Five

Toys, Technology, Gadgets and Gizmos

There are many devices available to make life easier and safer at home. I will share some of them with you in this chapter ranging from low tech to those more advanced and expensive systems.

1. **Motion and light detectors** to activate lights, appliances, etc.

   It is often helpful to activate lighting and appliances without having to find a switch. Great places for such a device include the workshop, laundry area, garage, and bathroom. There are several types of activators readily available in your local home improvement or hardware retailer, such as:

- Dusk to dawn detectors activate lights that remain on until dawn. They come in different configurations. Some can be screwed into an existing light fixture.
- Wall switches- these have to be installed into an existing wall switch and, if you're handy or know

of someone who is, they can be readily installed inexpensively.

- Self-standing detectors—I have found these units very handy in that they can activate a light or device when they detect motion or heat. They can be placed on the floor or table.

- In the laundry area and garage, I used a motion detector that easily screws into the light fixture and the bulb screws into it. Very handy and inexpensive.

These detectors and activators can be purchased from home improvement retailers and also from mail order catalogs like *Improvements* (1-800-642-2112) and www.safetyzone.com (see Bibliography).

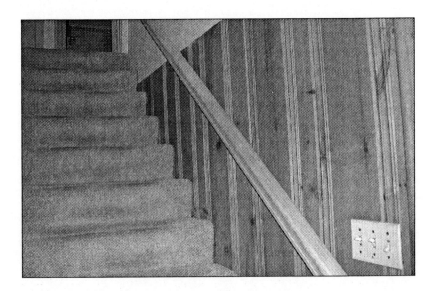

2. Railings for Stairways

When assessing stairways, there are various options to consider. One is to install (or rent) a stair glide, a moving chair device that rides on a railing on the stairs. These handy devices can negotiate turns and can be useful in handling groceries or supplies from the basement, for instance. If your stairway is narrow, install handrails on both sides of the stairway and make sure there is sufficient light and non-skid pads on the stairs themselves.

3. Railings for Walkways

When it became clear that my folks were having difficulty negotiating the hilly area of their backyard, I suggested a twenty-foot handrail. These are essential for difficult terrain or long stretches of walkway. My parents were very particular in the appearance of outdoor railing; hence, I used 2x2 pressure treated vertical pieces about 3 feet high with normal wooden deck railing for the horizontal rails. Coffee cans can convenient to use as cement bases, however, they do not last. There is specially designed cement for footings that should be used in whatever base you decide. In the ground, I have used wire mesh filled with stone, gravel upon which is poured the cement mix. Another alternative is to purchase preformed footings that are designed for above ground applications. Still another option is to install large metal "spikes" that secure a 4X4 piece of lumber. They come in two different lengths for different applications. These are useful for heavier applications, such as in water or where the depth is especially valuable. These spikes go into the ground farther than other options. I have great luck with them.

4. **Grab Bars** (vertical support in various styles and sizes)

There are various types, sizes and styles of Grab Bars. Select the one that satisfies the application intended. Two considerations to remember are the location of the device and the strength required for support. In some cases a simple oak towel bar might work well....looks nice and yet provides sufficient support for simple application where the risk of injury is low. These towel bars are attractive and, with some nails or screws to reinforce them, can provide decent support in non-safety applications. (Again, this creative approach would NOT be appropriate for a stairway where extra care and reliability of the device is critical for safety.) Be careful how the bar itself is attached to the wall. Some towel bars use light weight screws that clip onto the back of the unit. They will not provide sufficient support and should not be used. Rod iron towel bars can provide upper strength and be attractive. Long screws should be drilled into a stud in the wall, if not a stud, molly bolts should work fine. Check with your local home improvement store for details.

5. Timers

Although we have discussed them earlier, they are low-tech devices that are great for both security reasons and convenience. My family uses them for decorative lighting (inside and out), to maintain a lived-in appearance for security reasons, and for convenience when entering the house at night. I advocate timers for the activation of room air purifiers and humidifiers when you prefer *not* to have them on all the time.

6. Specific devices for individuals with specific challenges

- Talking devices, such as clocks

- Doorbells with blinking lights for individuals who are hearing impaired.

7. Doorbells

Hearing the doorbell or chime is important. Try adding several chime or bell units throughout the home; preferably those that are moveable. Using the battery operated units outside is helpful when your parents are enjoying the outdoors in their yard. They will be able to hear if someone is at the door much easier with the chime or bell near them.

8. Door Locks

As we mentioned earlier, there are many types of entry locks, including remote key fob types that operate your garage door, your entry door and lights.

9. A Creative Application of a Holiday Light switch-

Is a light switch, fan, humidifier, dehumidifier or stereo difficult to reach to turn on or off? A foot switch on a long extension cord, usually sold during the holidays, is handy because it enables activation of a hard-to-reach lamp or appliance. The cost is under $4.00 for a switch with extension cord on it. Some switches come with numerous end plugs to activate several lamps and devices. These are slightly more expensive. For the price and benefit, this is a great deal and can save a lot of pain, suffering and expenses by preventing accidents or injuries.

In addition to timers and motion detectors, there are more advanced tools and gadgets available for the home. Like all other tools and home enhancements, they should be chosen *to match* the skill, abilities and budget of the individuals using them. I've listed a couple below.

Automated home systems can now provide superior management of whole house heating, air conditioning, lighting, appliances, etc. These controls are managed by a computer laptop from across the country or across the room. However, with the convenience and advanced capabilities comes a hefty price tag, especially when the items are new to the market.

Kitchen Appliances

As we know, technology changes by the minute. Therefore, it is best to check for yourself as to senior-friendly appliances in preparation for making any innovations or home improvements. In my experience, there are several key factors to consider when evaluating laundry or kitchen appliances. These factors include:

- **Accessibility:** Is the door to the oven, washer or dryer easily accessible by those who will use it? Some washers and dryers offer risers to raise the units to a more convenient height.

- **Visibility:** Are the dials and controls clearly visible and the lighting of the controls bright enough?

- **Safety:** Are the controls safely accessible to the user? For instance, on a stove top, are the controls at the rear of the unit where the resident must reach *across* potentially hot elements and pans/pots in order to make changes...or are they safely located on the front of the stove? Are there sharp corners or edges on the controls or the unit itself that could catch clothing? Are the stovetop elements *cool* to the touch, using the latest in halogen technology?

- **Practicality:** Is the unit well suited for the abilities of those for which it is intended? Sometimes advanced technology is great for boomers but too complicated and involved for seniors or those with disabilities.

One example of future technology[5] in the home is the ***Electrolux Kelvinator*** division's introduction of a bilingual **washer** that gives vocal commands and information including an alert when there is an operator error.

In the future, refrigerators will warn you when milk is going bad. Microwaves will share recipes with you as well as setting the correct cooking time for your dish.[6]

Many of the appliance manufacturers incorporate valuable safety and convenience features; and as technology advances, consumers will have a better selection of safe and convenient appliances. (Two good sources for updated information are *Home and Garden television* and their website: www.hgtv.com and www. hometoys.com)

The Mealtime Kitchen[7] is a pilot program of the ***Internet Home Alliance*** committed to the merger of technology with convenience for homemakers. This non-profit consortium includes major manufacturers, such as IBM, Whirlpool, Sears, Icebox and Hewlett-Packard, that are all collaborating to enhance home appliances by using the latest technology. We're talking about advanced communication between the user and the appliance as well as appliance to appliance. For instance, a computer can save lives by reading labels on medicines and detecting possible interactions. The computer would then alert the owner or patient of a possible problem.

Some resources for more information about helpful devices:

- www.livinghome.com – look for Tech Homes.
- www.BeAtHome.com an Internet based home automation, services and security system starting at about $900 plus a monthly fee. Examples of services and capabilities provided include: monitoring the laundry room for leaks, ordering groceries on line, adjusting the thermostat and water heater, and managing all lights.
- www.hometoys.com This company publishes a newsletter and organizes national conferences pertaining to advance technology for the home. A perfect *boomer* site!

Chapter Six

Do-It-Yourself Innovations

So far, we've explored both subtle and obvious home enhancements that will enable your family members to live safer and more comfortable lives. This section covers some of the more creative aspects of this support.

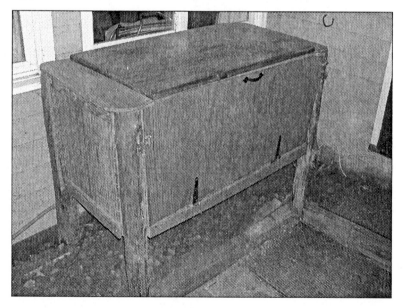

Storage bin (multi-function)

Let's admit it. We don't like to grow old and we don't want to be treated or thought of as an "elderly person" who requires special care. Here is an interesting story--

In *"The Oakes Homestead"*, there is a precarious step between the outside cooking area and the garage. Although the step will be replaced, it was obvious, when I noticed it, that some assistance (handrail) would be appropriate. I suggested that a handy horizontal handrail would help. My Mom responded that it would be too institutional. (Something that *old people* would use!). (Being undaunted I replied.)   ..."*How about a convenient, waist-high, elevated, rustic storage bin to be used for a work space (potting plants, etc.) in addition to storage*?" That creative idea was accepted. I subsequently designed and constructed this rustic, waist-high storage bin with the ability to be opened from the top or front. It turned out to be really handy, for working space as well as for storage. But the best of all, I have since noticed that my parents use it *for support* up the precarious steps! (They now have a storage bin....and a discreet, stylish support device!)

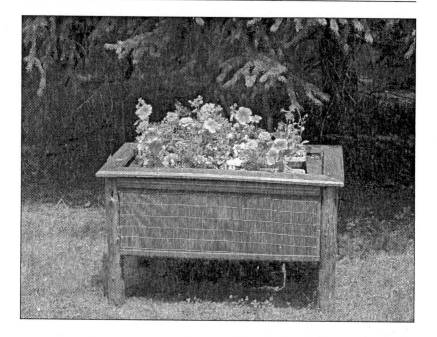

Convertible Planter Box (with hidden storage)
I designed a waist-high, elevated rustic planter that is
convertible. It serves as a decorative, functional planter
with space for planter inserts in the top, but it also can
be covered with a customized lid to enable it to be used
as a table. It has a hidden storage space for items, such
as plant spray, telephone, security device or even stereo
for discreet garden ambiance. (When the birds aren't
around, you bring your own bird sounds…with perhaps
a little Mozart all hidden behind burlap cloth sides.)

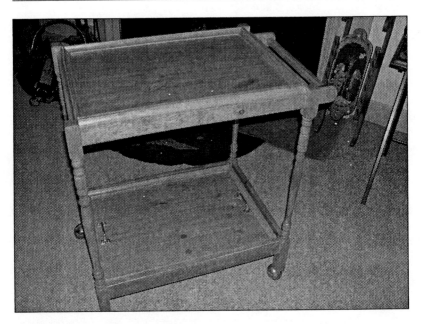

Teacart (multi-function)

With regard to inside mobility, I noticed that both my parents were experiencing some problems with walking in the house. Although they have become acclimated with the use of canes outside the house and at the market, they simply could not adjust to using them inside the home. Upon further discussion, we decided that a teacart of some type could help add walking stability and be practical at the same time. My subsequent research turned up empty. Nothing available on the market was reasonably priced and those I found did not blend into the style of my parent's home.

The solution: a customized teacart (insert) that provides stability and style. I made it to my Mom's size and needs. The lower shelf is removable allowing her to bring the cart close to her so it can be used as a workspace for writing or reading. The design allows for modifications for outdoor use.

Chapter Seven
Feng Shui for the Folks, Enhancing Home and Garden

This is my favorite chapter. This is when the fun begins! After the railings, hand holds and ramps are installed to protect and preserve…now let's work on improving the quality of life through enhanced ambiance and surroundings.

As I shared my thoughts on this chapter with a friend, she mentioned that a great deal of what I intended to share involves aesthetics and surroundings. To her it sounded like *Feng Shui* techniques. As I reflected on it, I agreed.

If you are unaware of the philosophy of Feng Shui, here is a brief overview.

Feng Shui, pronounced *"Fung Shway"*, revolves around the idea that energy management is the key to health, wealth and happiness. This energy, or "Chi", is needed to sustain all life. Feng Shui is the practice and study of directing energy through our homes and workspaces emphasizing the placement of furniture and utilization of water, metal, wood, fire and earth. Hence, the focus on windows, light sources, water features, wind chimes, etc.

(Source: www.fengshui.nabaza.org)

We are sensory beings who are influenced a great deal by our surroundings. Hence, as we strive to create positive, supportive environments for ourselves in our offices, homes and cars, it is useful to use all our senses as best we can. When working with our aging loved ones, our challenge is to accommodate diminished abilities and senses. Our sensory cells are aging as we do.

Using Aromas Makes *Scents!*

Aromas play an important part in our lives, both in protecting us and in enjoyment of life. The ability to detect rotting food or spoiled milk is important. On the more appealing side, the use of potpourri, aromatic candles and nebulizers can add a welcome dimension to the home. It is worth noting that lit candles can present a safety concern; therefore, electric atomizers and nebulizers can provide safe aromas without the dangers of using heat or flame. One source I have found helpful is the Leyden Co. (800-754-0668) for home air "enhancement" systems that include customized oils and nebulizers. Studies have shown that aromas can affect our mood and attitude. It's worth a try. After all, who can resist the smell of freshly baked breads or cookies? However, be sensitive that not everyone enjoys the aroma of rose, cinnamon, balsam or vanilla in whatever forms they take. Some people have allergies that limit their enjoyment and tolerance of aromas. Have fun doing some research if you have time. Certain scents affect people differently. For instance, vanilla and its derivatives can relax us while cinnamon and pine tend to stimulate us.

A sampling of some scents[8] and their benefits:

Lavender	Commonly used in Europe to scent linen closets and to control insects.	Peaceful, calming and stress-relieving
Bergamot	Leaves are used in Earl Grey tea. Even the roots are aromatic.	Used to combat depression and Seasonal Affective Disorder, SAD

Rose	The most expensive variety of oil comes from the Black Sea area, known as the Valley of the Roses.	Uplifting, serves to fight depression.
Vanilla	From the orchid family. The finest beans grown in Madagascar.	Fragrance used to calm and comfort.
Sweet orange	The plant is become a symbol of innocence and fertility.	Uplifting and clean-smelling.
Balsam	From evergreen trees	Energizing and uplifting.
Jasmine	Used frequently to greet guests in India.	Used to restore productive feelings and also fight depression.
Ylang Ylang	Used by sex therapists in Europe and in Indonesia.	Believed to be an aphrodisiac with its intensely sweet fragrance.
Rosewood	Taken from the wood chips of mature rosewood trees.	Believed to help stabilize the nervous system and help with regaining emotional balance.

Background Sounds and Music

As sensory beings, we respond to our surroundings through our senses. Our hearing enables us to detect threats. It also enables us to enjoy the sweet music of a flute, violin or waterfall. When enhancing the home of our parents, remember their abilities and preferences. Using music and sounds as environmental enhancements to *direct and manipulate* my mood, I create my own space to suit the particular effect I wish to enjoy at the moment. Whatever the desired effect, I put the suitable CD on my stereo and "ride the wave". As for my parents, they are experiencing hearing decline, especially in the higher frequencies of the spectrum. Therefore, I try to be sensitive as to the placement of speakers in the room so as not to impede conversation but to provide background music, as they choose. As for music, I have selected music they prefer and in lieu of their selection, I choose music to create the desired mood. In most cases, they like soft sounds of classical standards, or those of the Big Band era. However, they also enjoy Perry Como and the Kingston Trio. I have found that instruments they hear and enjoy tend to be of the mid-range frequency, for instance, vibes, piano, French horn and guitar.

Reminder: while sounds and music can enhance our lives, they can be distractions and impede communication and "connecting" with others.

Televisions and many portable stereo systems have timers on them. These can help in times of insomnia.

By the way, music and television can serve as inexpensive security systems when out of the house. Leaving them on does not take much electricity but offers a very real deterrent to would-be burglars. When gone at night, leave the radio or television on in a room with a light on to give the illusion of someone at home.

Waterfalls and Splashing Sounds
(avoid tinkling sounds)

For many of us, the soothing sound of splashing, gurgling and other water movement can be therapeutic. Outside, there are numerous possibilities to enhance your yard with a water feature. Only your imagination and budget limit you. My family has a 12-foot goldfish pond, which they enjoy during the good weather. In their enclosed patio, which is heated to a constant 50 degrees F in the winter, I created a temporary 3 foot pond that enables us to retain some of the outside water plants that would not otherwise survive outdoors during the winter. Together with automatic lighting, a small fountain and fogger, it provides a nice calm spot that is visible from inside the house. This retreat also provides a welcome escape for lunch on warmer winter days. The small fogger unit provides humidity to houseplants and the air in your home. When designing water features for seniors, be mindful that the sound of tinkling water (as from a steady stream of water) can suggest trips to the bathroom. Try using a small *waterwall* or water cascade. As always, be sensitive to the abilities of those utilizing these ideas. For the hearing impaired, waterfeatures can impede communication.

"Points of Color" Inside and Out

Whether inside or outside, visual stimulation can be appealing and gratifying. Again, you must remember the preferences and abilities of your parents as you design your overall strategy.

My family loves the outdoors and finds comfort and energy there. Special care is therefore taken to maintain and create a supportive and visually appealing backyard. "The Oakes Homestead" is on a lake with gazebo, goldfish pond and gardens.

Looking Out from Inside the House

The indoor heated patio offers a fabulous place to bring the outdoors indoors during the bleak midwinter. In the summertime, the air-conditioned patio provides a safe and healthy place to enjoy the summer and view outdoor gardens from a cool distance. Now come the challenges, as my parents continue to experience a decline in mobility and visibility. This inside display can be viewed from the kitchen or dining room. Location is important for maximum enjoyment all year long.

Outside in the Yard
(see back cover picture of a planter)

Bug and insect bite protection and prevention:
With West Nile Virus a possibility from mosquito bites, it is essential that we protect ourselves and our loved ones from bites and stings. Outdoor foggers and electronic gadgets can be of help and there are many options, both high and low tech. It seems that everyday a new device or product is on the market to prevent bites and stings. An important consideration: any one with a vision problem

should never use sprays, especially bug repellents! I have found the use of **bug repellent wipes** is really handy and helpful…and safe for use by visually impaired people. Obviously, using a spray can be harmful because you don't know where the spray will go, unless sprayed onto a cloth before applying to skin; hence, the benefit of these wipes. There are several manufacturers of these little wonders. A great idea.

There are now **Points of Color** throughout the backyard that are visible from the comfort of the inside patio. These areas of color concentration are numerous planter boxes of various sizes filled with vibrant colors that are seen from the house. So even when it's raining or too hot to be outside, they can enjoy the color of the season by looking out to the gardens.

Here are some tips for the garden:
- Use good **moisture retention potting soils** that include fertilizer and disease prevention additives. The soil is somewhat more expensive with these attributes, but in the long run, it will be worth it by producing healthier plants that will need less watering.

- In planters, use liners to preserve water and reduce maintenance during the summer.

- Try planting in **interchangeable planter boxes**. When using planter boxes of the same size, you can interchange them to suit the plant (if a plant likes more or less light in one area) or for a different look in the garden once in awhile.

- When possible, plant in *waist-high* **planters** for easy maintenance. Having the planters at this height will be more convenient and comfortable for seniors to maintain.

- Outside faucets can be difficult to reach, especially for your aging parents. For a low-cost solution, I have attached a **wire tomato "cage"** to the faucet that serves as both an extension and an easy way to turn the water on and off. The "cage" serves as a large steering wheel mechanism and while it may look peculiar, it can help. Word of caution: be sure the cage is attached securely to the faucet so that the water can be completely turned off.

- Lighting your outside garden for night enjoyment is nice, however, if you leave your blinds open at night, your home security could be compromised. You never know who might be looking into your home.

Therefore, it is suggested that you keep your blinds and shades closed at night. Also for security reasons, keep your shrubs trimmed back from the house so as not to allow would be burglars the protection they need while they break into your house.

- For security reasons, make sure shrubs near the house are trimmed back from the house so as not to allow would-be burglars protection while they break into your house. Visibility under and around bushes is important to see anyone standing behind the bushes.

- For easy maintenance, explore the possibility of **automated watering systems** for lawns and gardens. There are numerous types of systems ranging from drip style to major lawn irrigation arrangements. I can remember when my grandparents had a sprinkler that wheeled itself around the yard to water the lawn. Today, this gadget is still available and when combined with a timer, it is both inexpensive and quite handy. There are inexpensive faucet timers that can help manage your watering when you, the caregiver, are not available. Reminder: automation is not always received well by seniors. This new reliance on automation can be accompanied by a perceived loss of control. Your parents may simply decline the *automated* idea.

Outdoor Holiday Lighting

Lighting around the holidays can lift the spirits during the winter months. Holiday lighting can also send positive messages to neighbors that your aging parents are "still with the program" and "in the game". This positive message is also sent to the community with a well maintained home that is visible by neighbors. Again, a well-maintained home sends a message to would-be burglars that the residents care for their home and maintain (and protect) it!

Mobility Challenges

As for the **mobility challenge**, I purchased a reconditioned three-wheeled scooter for my Mom. No, not the kind your kids use. These are very advanced mobility units that can enable one or even two adults to get around in and outside their homes easily. Now my Mom can enjoy the garden and *points of color* up close and personal! Before the scooter, her mobility around the yard was difficult and her reduced vision frustrated her even more. Maintaining connections is important. Connecting with our environment, gardens, people and objects that make us feel secure, safe and content.

Outdoor Pathway

Speaking of connections, this spring my parents were experiencing difficulties getting down a hill in the backyard to their lakeside gazebo. Our yards change over time, as we do. The tree roots and grassy areas have become bumpy and rather dangerous for walking. One option is to root-prune and rid us of the obstacles. This option proved very strenuous and involved. (Chopping roots could damage or kill trees and shrubbery; creating more problems.) Of the various options we discussed, my parents and I decided on the construction of a 15-foot pathway *over* the roots. This path would be visually appealing, discreet and functional. My experience with a state park came in handy. The first thing we evaluated was the degree of abilities and challenges of my parents. In my case, my Father uses a walker, while my Mother uses the scooter. This path was subsequently constructed with these abilities in mind.

The materials included:

- Weed barrier cloth to reduce maintenance and prevent weeds from growing through our walkway.
- Pressure treated lumber for borders on both sides of the path.

- "Stone dust" gravel provided a fine and secure walking area; three inches deep.
- The handrails were made from pressure treated deck railings and supported by narrow, banister-type vertical pieces placed in cement bases. The handrails were on one side only. My parents opted not to use 4X4 supports, therefore, I used the smaller, banister type vertical pieces but supported by braces cemented into the ground at an angle.
- Cement was used as footings for the vertical pieces of the handrails and at select places on the walkway for added traction and to prevent washouts from water.
- Planter boxes can provide both visual guidance and attractive appeal when used as borders for the path. **Total cost =under $300.00** A great savings if you are willing to do the work yourself.

Healthy homes and house plants

Homes that are tightly sealed and insulated for energy savings can cause some problems with air quality. One of the best ways to cleanse the air in your home is by using plants. Two to three plants in 8-10 inch pots for every 100 square feet of space will help improve air quality. If you use more plants, it will take a shorter amount of time to improve the air and maintain a healthy home. Consider placing these plants near living spaces such as computer areas or near the television. While utilizing nature's way of cleaning the air with plants, remember that some people have allergies. Be sensitive and avoid making assumptions when it comes to making additions, changes or other modifications to your parent's home.

Some examples of nature's air purifiers include[9]:
- Bamboo palm
- Lady palm
- Dwarf date palm
- Janet Craig dracaena
- English ivy
- Kimberly queen
- Weeping fig
- Gerbera daisy
- Corn plant
- Warneckei dracaena

For more information:

- *How to Grow Fresh Air—50 Houseplants that Purify Your Home or Office*, Dr. B. C. Wolverton
- Plants for Clean Air Council's Web site: *www. plants4cleanair.org.*

Chapter Eight

Financial Considerations

As we know, aging and its consequences can be challenging in many ways. Although this text concentrates on making the home safe, secure and friendly for seniors, there are some pointers I'd like to share with you regarding reimbursements and other financial considerations.

It seems that almost daily there are many news stories about retirement, aging and financial planning. It's a concern to many baby boomers and seniors alike, as you and I both know. Unfortunately, seniors can become victims of scams and abuse by individuals and corporations. The other day there was a story on the news about the disclosure of fees and costs associated with financial planners and related services. Fees and related costs can be hidden and sometimes misleading. When you're looking for a Financial Planner or reviewing the existing one of your parents, it's good to investigate the fee structure and their compensation method. I have found that Financial Planners are compensated in two ways, commissions on transactions and percentage of the total value of the portfolio. It's in your best interest to become aware of how your Planner is paid because it reflects how they are motivated. The way a person is compensated usually is connected to the way they are motivated.

Medicare will not pay for devices or home improvements that are *NOT medically essential.*

For instance, **walk ramps** outside of your house are not covered. **Scooters** used *inside* the home may be covered but if used only outside the house, they are not. **Electric stair glides** (chairs on tracks that enable individuals to *glide* up and down the stairs in/or outside the home) are *not* covered. The reasoning…if the resident *needs* to go into the basement of their home and cannot do so, they should move. For more information and clarification, contact Medicare at: 1-800-633-4227 or www.medicare.gov.

Long Term Care Insurance

If you purchase long-term care insurance, some of these policies cover home care that is provided by family caregivers. I suggest you check it out.

Reverse Mortgages

Most seniors are concerned about financial security and the ability to maintain a healthy cash flow. One solution is something called a "reverse mortgage". Essentially, if you own a condo or house, a reverse mortgage enables you to treat the equity in your home as a source of funds for your use. Upon the sale of the property, the net profits would reflect the amount of funds drawn from the original value of the property. So, if cash flow is of concern and you own property, you should investigate reverse mortgages.

Chapter Nine

Security Scams and Seniors

The avoidance of scams requires knowing where to report suspicious proposals and contracts, where to go for more information and overall vigilance. Seniors often fall prey to unscrupulous vendors, contractors, financial planners and other service personnel. In my judgement, seniors are more often vulnerable because they tend to be more trusting. Today, unfortunately, everyone must be suspicious about things we read, hear and see.

There are many suspicious deals and offers to avoid. This chapter is designed to highlight some personal experiences and offer some suggestions. Further research and investigation would be advised.

To date, my family has avoided being taken or scammed. In my role as son and caregiver, I will continue to do all I can to protect them.

Example

A gentleman, with a wad of bills, drove through my folks' neighborhood and knocked on doors and introduced himself as an "Antique Appraiser". (Funny, he wasn't that old to be referred to as "*antique*".) Apparently, he had neither town permit nor permission of the community association to solicit door to door. (Many private communities post their policy on public soliciting.) Nonetheless, trusting residents invited this person into their homes to "assess" their valuables. He made some purchases on the spot. I had the following concerns:

1. He had no permit
2. He had no permission from the private community to go door to door
3. He could have been assessing more than antiques. He could have been evaluating burglary possibilities and could return later for a break-in.

I was later advised by the Police Department that vendors and solicitors who are not selling anything, do NOT require permits in town! So even without a permit, these strangers can legally solicit in neighborhoods (that allow it), leaving residents potentially exposed to fraud and crime. Find out what your community allows!

Common ways that outsiders can infiltrate or penetrate the home:

1. Mail

- We all receive tons of unsolicited mail daily. Much of it is from charities seeking donations. Once you give to one charity, it will not only solicit from you more often, but also they will probably share your address with others. Consequently, defining which charities you will support and *ignoring all others* can drastically reduce this "junk mail".

2. Phone

- The use of phone message machines can enable you to screen out incoming phone calls. However, these machines can also prevent emergency contact and therefore may not be recommended in all instances. For instance, the use of a *First Alert* system requires the ability of the service to contact you and if you don't respond, they will react accordingly with emergency personnel. If you use an answering machine, this may impede the effectiveness of this aspect of their service.

- Many people are trusting and therefore gullible and vulnerable on the phone to callers. No one should ever provide confidential, personal information on the phone unless you are familiar with the caller and the organization, such as a doctor.

Example

Although there is a national no-call listing to reduce the number and nuisance of telemarketing to homes, non-profit organizations can contact you. When I received a call some months ago, I was asked to contribute to some police-related charity. Whether legitimate or not, there are some precautions to take when you are called. I questioned the caller, "How do I know you *are* who you propose to be? I need some proof of your identity and authenticity." I continued with, "What percentage of the contribution actually is received by the charity? Send me collateral material and I will consider it."
Many telemarketers will want you to remain on the call for further discussion and perhaps will even debate you on issues pertaining to their cause. In many cases, they are professional telemarketers and really not committed to any cause but making money for themselves!

3. Computer/Internet
- Technology is amazing. However, it can also enable criminals to access personal data via your phone line into your computer, not to mention

the exposure to viruses from the Internet. The investment in software such as McAfee and Norton Systems can be well worth the cost.

4. **Identity theft** is a major concern today. Without becoming paranoid, there are some basic preventive measures to take:

- Avoid exposing your confidential information to anyone by word or documents. Be sure to buy a shredder and use it to destroy sensitive information before throwing it in the garbage. This sensitive information includes bank account numbers, social security identification and credit card identification. Also, shred credit card solicitation with your "pre-approved" number on it. I have heard stories how these can be used to assume your identify and rack up some serious bills in *your name!*

AARP has the following tips to prevent identify theft[10]:

- Never share your Social Security number or other personal information to anyone over the phone or email unless you initiate the contact.
- Shred all documents that have your confidential information and account numbers on them *before* disposing of the documents.

- Use a locked mailbox or the post office to mail checks.
- Review your personal credit reports periodically to make certain that there are no surprises there, such as an address change.
- Review your bank statements carefully for suspicious activity.
- When using your bank's automated teller machines, be careful that no one is close by to view personal information and passwords.
- When using a computer at home, install firewall security software to further protect your personal information on the PC.
- Private Identification Numbers (PIN) should be memorized and not written down. If you must write them down, be careful where you store them.

5. Contractors and outside vendors
Some pointers on how to prevent scams from home improvement contractors[11]:
- Avoid all pressure decision timelines from contractors, such as *"Today only..."*
- Get three quotations.
- Get references from local customers.

- Have a knowledgeable contact review contracts before signing.
- Ask for a certificate of insurance for the proposed work. This document verifies that you are covered in event of mishaps on the job.
- Call the Department of Consumer Protection (in CT 800-842-2649) and the Better Business Bureau (CT 203-269-2700) to learn of any problems or complaints on file involving the contractor.
- You have the right to cancel the contract. Even if you have signed a contract, you have the right to cancel without penalty within the following three business days.

Example

My parents once scheduled a home visit with an insurance salesperson to present a long term care insurance policy. I became uncomfortable when it was evident that my folks were taking this gentleman's word that he was who he said he was! When I became suspicious and asked for credentials and that material be sent to me prior to the meeting, he became defensive and uncooperative! A phone call to the local Police Department proved helpful. They were willing to have a cruiser park at the end of the driveway during the meeting. Although I appreciated this generous offer, I canceled the meeting. While this may sound rather paranoid, you cannot be too trusting today. We tell our children not to speak to strangers. This same precaution should be taken with seniors. Being too trusting can prove fatal!

Misplaced trust can become disastrous.

For more information and to report problems, contact your local and state authorities, including the Better Business Bureau, the Consumer Affairs Department and the Department of Aging.

Additional contacts involving security and identify protection:

American Institute of Philanthropy
4579 Laclede Avenue, Suite 136
St. Louis, MO 63108-2103
314-454-3040

National Charities Information Bureau
19 Union Square West, 6th floor
New York, New York 10003-3395
212-929-6300
Philanthropic Advisory Service Council of the Better Business Bureaus
4200 Wilson Boulevard, Suite 800
Arlington, VA 22203-1838
703-276-0100

Direct Marketing Association
Telephone Preference Service
P.O. Box 9014
Farmingdale, NY 11735-9014

Federal Trade Commission
Boston Regional Office
101 Merrimac Street, Suite 810
Boston, MA 02114-4719
617-424-5960

Chief Postal Inspector –Postal Crime Hotline
475 L'Enfant Plaza, SW, Room 3100
Washington, DC 20360
202-268-4298 or -4299

FBI's Internet Fraud Complaint Center:
www.ifccfbi.gov
Identity Theft Resource Center:
www.idtheftcenter.org
Privacy Rights Clearinghouse:
www.privacyrights.org
Free handbook from the Federal Trade Commission:
"ID Theft: When Bad Things Happen to Your Good Name"
www.ftc.gov/bcp/coline/pubs/credit/idtheft.htm   or
call AARP at: 888-687-2277

If you suspect identity theft, contact the credit reporting
agencies and place a "fraud alert" on your accounts.
• Equifax: 888-766-0008 or www.equifax.com
• Experian: 888-397-3742 or www.experian.com
• TransUnion: 800-680-7289 or www.transunion.com
• Federal Trade Commission: 877-438-4338

Bibliography and Handy Resources

Organizations, associations and other resources

Children of Aging Parents, CAPS

www.caps4caregivers.org

A non-profit organization whose mission is to assist the nation's nearly 54 million caregivers of the elderly or chronically ill with reliable information, referrals and support. CAPS is a member of Independent Charities of America. 1609 Woodbourne Road, Suite 302A, Levittown, PA 19057 800-227-7294

AARP

1-888-OURAARP (687-2277) Mon-Fri 8-8 ET   601 E. Street NW, Washington, DC 20049 www.aarp.org

National Resource and Policy Center on Housing and Long Term Care

www.aoa.dhhs.gov/Housing/modifications.html.

CareGuide 1-888-389-8839

www.careguide.com An award-winning site of resources, referral network, care providers, services, articles, interviews and other helpful information. They provide management of care for loved ones usually through an employer's Employee Assistance Program (EAP); however, they do provide "retail" services...for a fee.

Agencies and Associations

Great resources for information, facts and research.

Medicare

1-800-633-4227 Available 24 hours a day TTY users should call 1-877-486-2048 www.medicare.gov

Administration on Aging—Elders & Families:
www.aoa.gov/eldfam.asp

Alzheimer's Association:
 www.alz.org

American Association of Homes and Services for the Aging:
 www.aahsa.org

Caregivers & Companions:
www.caregivershome.com

Centers for Medicare and Medicaid Services:
www.medicare.gov
ElderCare Location:
www.eldercare.gov
Family Caregiver Alliance:
www.caregiver.org
National Alliance for Caregiving:
www.caregiving.org (presents reviews of web sites, videos, newsletters and more.)
National Council on the Aging:
www.ncoa.org
National Family Caregivers Association:
www.nfcacares.org
NOCA Benefits Checkup:
www.benefitscheckup.org
Taking Care of Yourself as a Caregiver:
www.careguide.com
Today's Caregiver:
www.caregiver.com (discussion forum and links)
U.S. Administration on Aging:
www.aoc.gov

Retail Sources catalogs of helpful devices and gadgets

HSN Catalog Service, Inc.

Patrickf@hsn.net 216-831-6191 X 230

MaxiAids catalog

Products for independent living 800-522-6294

Independent Living Aids, Inc.

Can-Do Products for your active, independent life

1-800-537-2118 www.independentliving.com

Improvements

www.safetyzone.com 1-800-642-2112

Living Air

Electronic air purification systems 612-780-9388

9199 Central Avenue NE Blaine, MN 55434

Leyden Aromas

A great source for small to large air enhancement systems and nebulizers.

800-754-0668

The New England Assistive
Technology Marketplace (NEAT)

An information and resources service to individuals interested in various types of *assistive technology*. A fabulous resource.

1-866-525-4492, 860- 243-2869

Info@neatmarketplace.org

Vision Dynamics

A Connecticut retailer specializing in visual aids.

203-271-1944 www.visiondynamics.com

Books and Periodicals

Caring for Your Aging Parents

A complete guide for children of the elderly by Robert R. Cadmus, M.D. Prentice-Hall, Inc. Englewood Cliffs, New Jersey, 1984

The Complete Guide to Eldercare

A.J. Lee and Melanie Callender, Ph.D. Barron's Educational Series, Barron's, New York 1998

Aging Parents and You
A complete handbook to help you help your elders maintain a healthy, productive and independent life by Eugenia Anderson-Ellis. Marsha Dryan Master Media, New York, 1988

How to Care for Aging Parents by Virginia Morris, Workman Publishing, New York 1996.

Home Safety Guide for Older People :
Check It Out/Fix it Up by Jon Pynoos and Evelyn Cohen, Serif Press, Inc. 1331 H. Street NW, Washington DC 20005 202-737-4650

Safety for Older Consumers, U.S. Consumer Product Safety Commission, Washington D.C. 20207 1-800-638-2772 Free handbook

Other books on this topic:
- **How to Care for Aging Parents** by Virginia Morris and Robert Butler
- **The Complete Eldercare Planner:** Where to Start, Questions to Ask and How to Find Help by Joy Loverde

- **Coping With Your Difficult Older Parent:
  A Guide to Stressed-Out Children** by Grace
  Lebow, et al
- **Caring for Yourself While Caring for Your Aging
  Parents: How to Help, How to Survive** by Claire
  Berman

**Additional contacts involving security and identify
protection:**

American Institute of Philanthropy
4579 Laclede Avenue, Suite 136
St. Louis, MO 63108-2103
314-454-3040

National Charities Information Bureau
19 Union Square West, 6th floor
New York, New York 10003-3395
212-929-6300

Philanthropic Advisory Service Council of the Better
Business Bureaus
4200 Wilson Boulevard, Suite 800
Arlington, VA 22203-1838
703-276-0100

Direct Marketing Association
Telephone Preference Service
P.O. Box 9014
Farmingdale, NY 11735-9014

Federal Trade Commission
Boston Regional Office
101 Merrimac Street, Suite 810
Boston, MA 02114-4719
617-424-5960

Chief Postal Inspector –Postal Crime Hotline
475 L'Enfant Plaza, SW, Room 3100
Washington, DC 20360
202-268-4298 or -4299

FBI's Internet Fraud Complaint Center:
www.ifccfbi.gov
Identity Theft Resource Center:
 www.idtheftcenter.org
Privacy Rights Clearinghouse:
www.privacyrights.org

Free handbook from the Federal Trade Commission: *"ID Theft: When Bad Things Happen to Your Good Name"* www.ftc.gov/bcp/coline/pubs/credit/idtheft.htm or call AARP at 888-687-2277

If you suspect identity theft, contact the credit reporting agencies and place a "fraud alert" on your accounts.
* Equifax: 888-766-0008 or www.equifax.com
* Experian: 888-397-3742 or www.experian.com
* TransUnion: 800-680-7289 or www.transunion.com
* Federal Trade Commission: 877-438-4338

Parting Comments

As we close, I'd like you to revisit the picture on the cover. In addition to being a dedication to my parents, this shot says a lot. Upon closer inspection, you will find the following items in this tranquil setting:

- **A walking cane** – representing safety and security.
- **Windchimes** – symbolizing the appreciation and beauty of nature.
- **Colorful flowers** – emphasizing visual enlightenment and the benefits of flowers and plants.
- **Telephone holder** – reminds us of the importance of connection and communication among each other and those distant from us.
- Above all, there are two seniors enjoying quality time together in a peaceful and secure setting.

Aging is never convenient and presents many challenges for families and individuals. As children of aging parents, this is the time for us to support and love *them* the way they did us for so many years. There are many innovative tips and techniques you can apply, or create to help your loved ones remain in their own home. I hope they have inspired you to develop your own solutions and injury prevention techniques.

-Chuck Oakes

No device, gadget or gizmo will ever replace compassion and kindness towards one another.

Endnotes

[1] Metropolitan Life Insurance Company (1997). The MetLife study of employer costs for working caregivers. www.caregiving.org/metlife.pdf

[2] Source: CareGuide, www.careguide.com/CareGuide/ careathomecontentview see Bibliography and Resources

[3] Source: AARP

[4] Town of West Hartford, CT

[5] Residential Architect, April 2003, Nigel F. Maynard

[6] Successful Farming, March, 2002, Cheryl Tevis

[7] Cox News Service, Kitty Crider, Nov 25, 2003

[8] Aromatherapy for Health, Relaxation and Well-Being, Joanne Rippin, Lorenz Books, 1997 and Fragrant Herbal, Leslie Bremness, Bulfinch, 1998.

[9] Better Homes & Gardens, March 2002, Laura O'Neil:

[10] AARP Bulletin February 2004

[11] Source: www.arnieps.org

Printed in the United States
34588LVS00002B/141